Searching the Web
for Health

Searching the Web for Health

◆

A Guide to Finding Reliable Medical Information on the Internet

Gary Paul Bryant

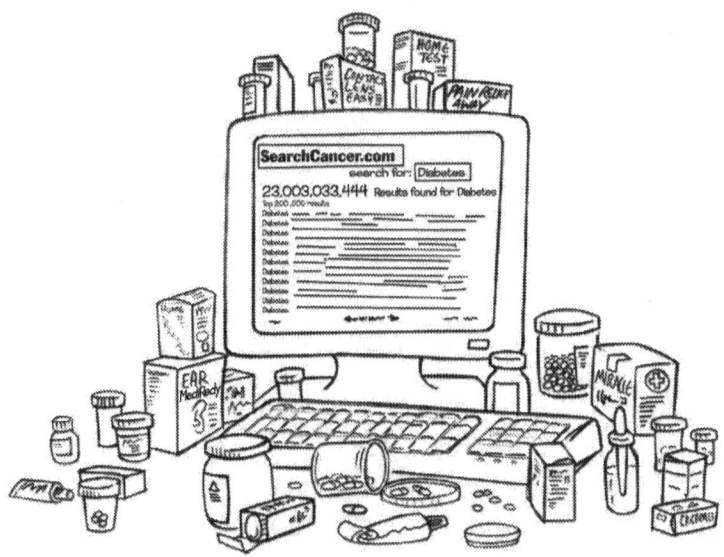

iUniverse, Inc.
New York Lincoln Shanghai

Searching the Web for Health
A Guide to Finding Reliable Medical Information on the Internet

iUniverse, Inc.

For information address:
iUniverse, Inc.
2021 Pine Lake Road, Suite 100
Lincoln, NE 68512
www.iuniverse.com

ISBN: 0-595-30343-9

Printed in the United States of America

Contents

Acknowledgements

Lou Knecht, Deputy Chief, Bibliographic Services Division, NLM, Washington, D.C.

Sabrina Crisp, Web Development, U.S. Food & Drug Administration, Washington, D.C.

Sandra Koopman-Bryant, R.N. CCRN, University of Washington, Seattle, Washington

Phil Holloway, Illustrator, Montreal, Quebec

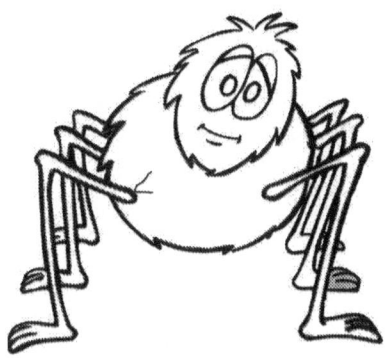

I. Introduction

Searching the Web for health information can be a daunting task. Even putting aside those Web pages that simply sell low cost drugs or magic elixirs, reliable information can be hard to come by. Worse still, it is nearly impossible to tell the difference between information you can use and information that really is not information at all.

Add to this the fact that medical information is complex. Hundreds of press announcements about new drugs and treatments are released everyday. Seemingly conflicting study results creep into the mainstream media, confusing us even further. Most of us do not have advanced degrees in bioengineering, chemistry, genetics or mathematics. Most of us cannot pronounce the name of our own prescriptions, never mind understand the inner workings of molecular relationships. Even our own doctors are subject to the same deluge of information. There are more patients, more costs, and less time. Mistakes will happen. Now, more than ever, it is crucial for us as consumers to understand modern medicine, and in so doing, to become partners in our own healthcare.

If you are like most people, you probably tried a search tool like Google or Yahoo to locate some kind of health information. You might have been curious about the diagnosis of a friend or, more likely, you have been diagnosed with something yourself, and you did not like what the doctor told you. So you go to your computer, type a few words into the search engine form, hit 'Enter', and in a few minutes you are faced with thousands of citations to sift through. After twenty or thirty minutes, you find that one page simply leads to another that leads to another. The answer to your original query is elusive. Even if you do find a page that looks promising, small text at the bottom indicates that it was last updated in 1997—hardly cutting edge technology.

To make matters worse, and better, new medical therapies and treatments *are* being developed for hundreds of diseases and conditions. Hidden among the advertorials for dubious home remedies and low cost pharmaceuticals from third-world countries, are solid pronouncements of real advances in medical science. That does not mean that every news release from a famous research institute signals the discovery of a cure for cancer or Alzheimer's disease. Many such releases simply provide information about new therapies that alleviate symptoms. The issue for us, as consumers, is locating this information, and that is where this book comes in.

We want to provide an easy-to-read tutorial for finding real medical information on the World Wide Web. We offer a review of the traditional search process and point out some of the important features of the Internet and how they relate to investigating medical issues on the Web.

Here you will find a big picture appraisal of how the medical and health industries employ Web technology, the role of commercial opportunism in this process, and how it can distort or hide the information you may be seeking.

In *Searching the Web for Health*, you will learn how Web pages are constructed and how that can affect your search results. Also included are software tools and search strategies that can save time and reduce the likelihood of your obtaining incorrect information.

We will discuss Web privacy and how to safeguard yourself during an online search. The names of important organizations, Web sites, and portals are provided as well as some perspective on where to get the latest medical news, how to find clinical trials, and where to locate institutions that are doing research on the health issues that interest you. Keep in mind that the Web sites we mention in this book are presented as examples of the points we will be discussing—they are not meant to be a complete list.

Thus, *Searching the Web for Health* is designed to assist health consumers in obtaining accurate medical information, to empower consumers and their families, and to help them become equal partners in decisions concerning their health.

WHAT THIS BOOK IS NOT

Searching the Web for Health is not a tutorial on Web technologies, Web programming, or software. It is not a primer for professional medical researchers. There is no discussion of standards for citations or document usage for professional researchers or editors. Most important, *Searching the Web for Health* is not intended to be used as a medical resource.

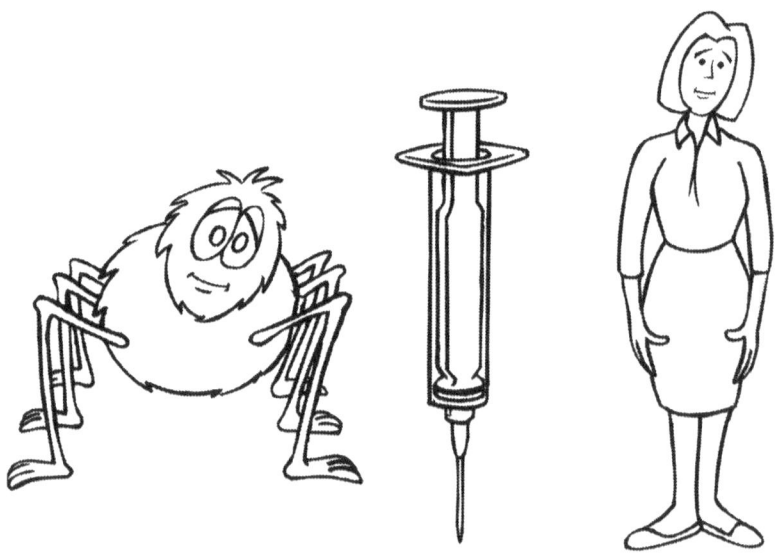

II. The Web, Medicine, and You

When it comes to your health, having the best information available is crucial. Unfortunately, the lure of the Web and its easy access can give consumers a false sense of power. Just tap in a few "key words" and there is the answer to our question, or so we think.

Although search engines do provide a definitive information service to Internet users, higher standards are crucial when it comes to medical information because misinformation can have real—possibly dire—consequences.

BROWSER BASICS

Since most of what we will be talking about is on the Internet, it would be a good idea to review the use of your Web browser. While some of this information may seem redundant, you may pick up a few tips to make your Web searching more efficient and rewarding.

YOUR BROWSER

Your browser is that piece of software that allows you to access Web pages on the Internet. While most people access the Web with some version of Microsoft's Internet Explorer, other browsers including Netscape, America Online (which uses an embedded version of Netscape), David Gay's Opera, and a few others remain viable alternatives.

Your browser can bring information to you in several ways. You can simply type in a Web address, known as a Universal Resource Location (URL),e.g., http://www.breakthroughdigest.com. You could also start from your default home page and begin clicking on links within the browser window.

'Plug-ins', small add-on pieces of software such as MacroMedia's Flash or Real Networks Real Player, can be downloaded to your system. Plug-ins allow you to view extended animations, listen to audio files, watch videos, and interact in other ways, using a wide variety of formats, and giving your browser functionality that it may not have had in its original configuration. Many plug-ins are preinstalled in newer browser versions.

ABOUT URLs

Here are a few common mistakes people make while using their Web browser. These mistakes can affect the quality of your search. First, the Web address.

Suppose you are at Google, and you click on a link that seems to be the answer to your Web hunting dreams. A few seconds later, one of two things happens. Either you find yourself viewing a rather simplistic Web page that screams 'File not found' or you arrive at page that is unrelated to your search.

With the 'File not found" screen you may still be able to find your information. Suppose, for example, the Web address was http://www.breakthroughdigest.com/this_is_the page.html. Try typing in only the domain name (i.e., the part of the Web address before the '/') like this—http://www.breakthroughdigest.com. Webmasters occasionally move files or re-organize their Web sites. If a Web site becomes too unwieldy or its content increases unexpectedly, the entire site may be reconfigured in a new way. The result is that existing information gets moved around, and the search engine or directory that you originally used to find the page does not yet reflect the changes.

By typing in the domain name only, you are likely to find the home page of the Web site that hosted your page. You can also use links from the web page menu to drill down through the links it provides to possibly find your information.

Sometimes Web sites simply run out of steam, shut down, or get bought by other companies. This can explain why you might arrive at a Web page advertising computers rather than a page displaying the medical report you were expecting to see. In these cases, Web administrators have 'redirected' the Web site address to the hosting company or new owner. If this is the case, you can assume that the Web page for which you were looking is no longer available.

NAVIGATING WEB SITES

Web sites can be as simple as a one-page html document that has some text and a few links. They can also be complicated, including frames, audio and video, interactive forms, and hidden codes that track your every click. There may be search boxes that allow you to search only the site you are visiting or you may be able to search the entire Web. Make sure you are aware of which type of Web site you are using.

As part of the research process, you will often have to scroll down long pages of lists. You can, however, save some time by using the 'find' feature. In Microsoft Explorer, for example, click on the 'edit' menu near the top left part of the browser. Scroll through the list of options and select 'Find on this page'. Using this tool, you can jump directly to the portion of the page that contains the key word(s) for your search. It really works!

RESEARCHING HEALTH INFORMATION

There are three things you will need to understand to facilitate your search for health information on the Web. They are:

- **Your Role as the Researcher**
  Before you begin your search, it is important to have a clear picture of your own motives and knowledge base. Remember: You are looking for real medical information, not product promotions or philosophical statements on magnetism or stone therapy.

- **How the Web works**

  You need to understand the various components of the Web, how they work together, and how technology and commercial forces affect the content of the information that is available to you.

- **How the Medical Industry Uses the Web**

  Finally, you need to understand how medical research gets published and why one medical story may make it to the CNN news report while another does not.

With an understanding of these issues as the foundation for a health information search, we can now look at some of the more effective ways of extracting the kind of information you are seeking.

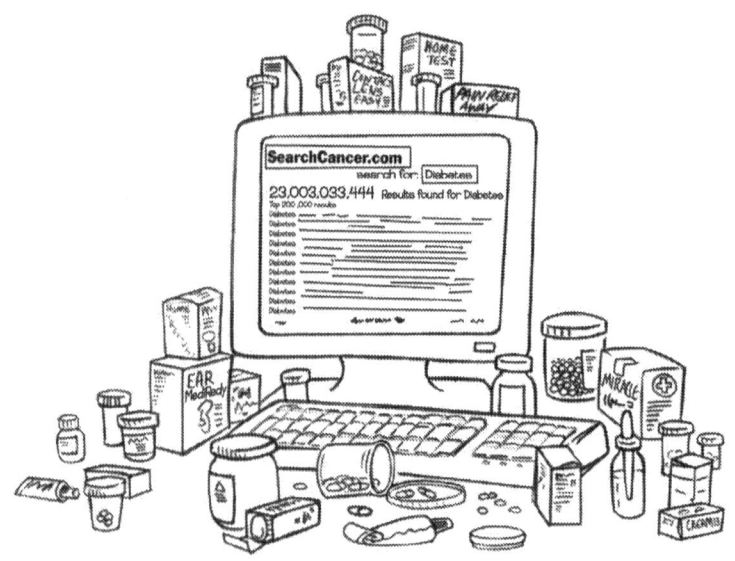

III. First, Search Yourself

The answer you get from any research attempt is only as good as the question you ask. Suppose, for example, you are looking for the latest treatment for Stargardt's Disease, but you spell it 'Stargard'. That mistake reduces exponentially your chances of finding the right information or even related information.

More important, what happens when you do find something of value? Will you recognize it when you see it? Before beginning a search, take time to evaluate your knowledge of the subject and any possible bias you may have for a particular search engine, treatment philosophy, or regimen. If you have any doubt about your expertise in the medical arena (and I hope you do), then you must start from scratch and pretend you no nothing about the subject of your inquiry. By starting fresh at the top of the soon-to-be-learned factoids, you can prepare yourself to ask the right questions. There are two steps to this process:

1. LEARN THE VOCABULARY

This is easier than you think. Well maybe not, but it is easier than *I* thought it would be. Learning a new vocabulary is all about acclimating. You need to be around those words a while to feel comfortable with them. You can do this by pointing your Web browser to http://www.eurekalert.org and browsing the thousands of medical press releases. Start by doing a search on the general topic you're interested in, maybe cancer or diabetes. Now use your Web browser and open a second window, point that browser window to http://www.healthfinder.gov. In the little search form at the top, type in the word 'glossary'. In a moment you will see about seventy medical glossaries listed in your search result. Find the one on cancer and you are set to go. While reading your press releases in one window, you can 'copy and paste' the terms you do not understand in the glossary window of HealthFinder.gov. Spend some time doing this, and you should get a better idea of the kinds of questions you should be asking.

2. GETTING UP-TO-SPEED ON YOUR SUBJECT

Part of your background investigation should include a review of the historical information surrounding your topic. Suppose, for example, you are researching diabetes. You will learn that there are two major types. One affects children, while the other, adult-onset type II diabetes, primarily affects adults. It is interesting to note that while both types lead to insufficient insulin production, diabetes, itself, develops in completely different ways. Thus, any intelligent query into new treatments or clinical trials will depend on how well informed you are about the disease itself. Do you want to know about type I diabetes or type II? Bone Up!

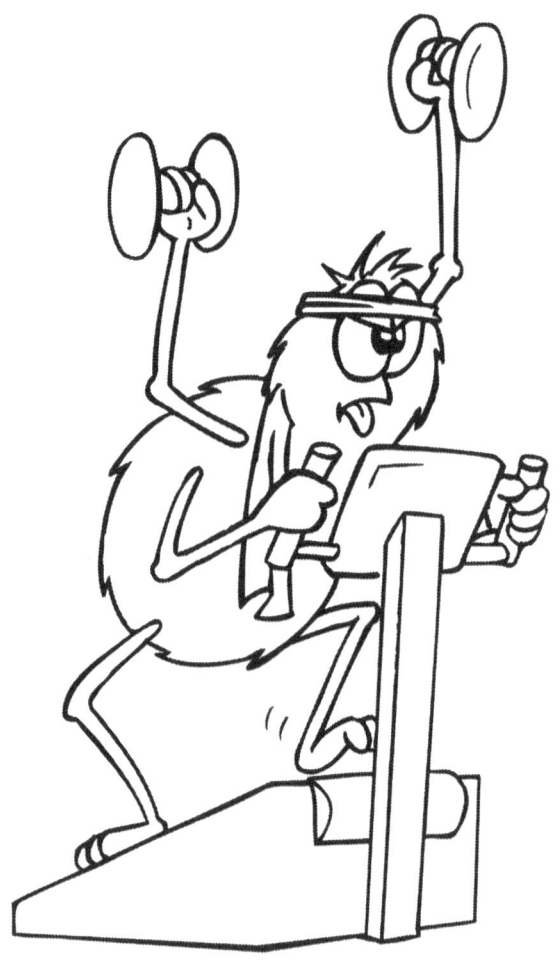

IV. The Healthy Web

The World Wide Web (or 'the Web') is only *one* part of the Internet. The Internet exists to deliver all kinds of information to all kinds of people through computers known as servers. These servers are connected by a variety of networks all over the world. If you have a computer and a modem, you are connected to one of these networks. The term 'World Wide Web was coined by Tim Berners-Lee, who is considered the originator of the Web. He is currently Director of the World Wide Web Consortium, which creates the standards by which the Web operates.

The World Wide Web is only one way of delivering information through the Internet. Internet components include E-mail, File Transfer Protocol (FTP), Telnet and Newsgroups among others. What makes the Web so special is its ability to make some of those other Internet features available through a Web browser and, more important, its ability to link to related documents. This linking is referred to as *hypertext*.

Hypertext is the concept behind the Hyper Text Markup Language (HTML), which is the original script language of Web pages. Anytime you click on a link, you are using hypertext. Other Web scripting languages such as ASP, XHTML, PHP, etc., have improved on the original HTML, but the principles of content association based on hypertext remain unchanged.

THE WEB IS IMPORTANT

According to the Computer Industry Almanac, there will be more than 945 million Internet users by 2004. In the United States, Nielsen/NetRatings puts the number of Internet users at 165.7 million in 2002, out of a total U.S. population of 280.5 million.

Virtually every political entity from government offices, to state, city, and county administrations are connected (or connecting) to the Internet. Every college and university, every major corporation, and most small businesses have an Internet presence in some form. The Web has become a part of modern life for most of us and is affecting the lives of nearly everyone.

HEALTH RESEARCH ON THE WEB: BE VERY SKEPTICAL

There is a lot of health related content on the Web. Much of what you will find by searching Google, Yahoo, and other search engines will be, at best, unconfirmed, and possibly even dangerous if you act on it without checking its authenticity and consulting your doctor. There are several reasons for this and it is important that you understand why we find ourselves in a situation where we have lots of information but little useful knowledge.

ANYONE CAN CREATE A WEB PAGE, OR CAN THEY?

Almost every Internet access account comes with a mechanism to create your own Web page. Some users have never bothered to create a Web site, while others have developed elaborate Web sites with all kinds of content. Since there is no enforcement agency governing Web publishing, the Web is a hodgepodge of facts and fantasy. In terms of medical and health content, we see everything from research findings from leading institutions to anecdotal tirades by unhappy recipients of any given treatment.

There are electronic forums where any user can post an authoritative claim about some aspect of health research. Commercial enterprises often emphasize certain aspects of legitimate research findings while diminishing the implications of other findings. And then there are the growing number of advertorials, the clever melding of a commercial sales pitch with kernels of real knowledge are designed to persuade you to buy a particular product.

THERE ARE NO LAWS REGULATING HOW INFORMATION IS POSTED

As we have noted, there are no laws governing how web pages are published. Because any motivated individual can produce a convincing Web site, regardless of the source of content, your research must include a way to establish the authenticity of Web site content BEFORE you make a decision about how you will use that information.

Several organizations are attempting to develop standards for health content on the Web. Links to these organizations are included in the resource section of this book.

Plagiarism is Rampant on the Web

Plagiarism, i.e., the unauthorized copying of copyrighted material, is a special consideration on the Web. With regard to health-related content, this is particularly important for three reasons:

1. Unqualified content providers can misrepresent their expertise by including unauthorized information on their own site.

2. There is no way that consumers can be sure that all material has been included in its entirety.

3. Plagiarism is, quite simply, illegal.

Web Sites are Either Not Maintained or are Poorly Maintained

While it is easy to throw up a Web site, maintaining that Web site is time consuming and potentially costly. Even for large institutions, outdated Web content, broken hyperlinks, and poor page formatting add another level of frustration to the search for health information on the Web. Lack of consistent publishing standards in the industry is a major barrier to accessing reliable information.

Web Content Does Not Expire

Timing is everything, which is why the Web is a leading medium for delivering breakthrough news and information. You can get it right now. The downside is that you can probably see the exact same news page in 5 years because much of it is not dated and most of the outdated material is never removed. It is important to remember, then, that the information you find on the Web may not be the very latest and most up to date.

COMMERCIALIZATION OF THE SEARCH ENGINES HAS AFFECTED SEARCH RESULTS

The integration of paid listings into search results has become an increasing problem over the past couple of years. Because of the difficulty of maintaining revenues from banner advertising, many search engines and directories have developed 'position based' preferential listings for Web site owners willing to pay for the privilege of being listed higher in the search engine result page. Suppose, for example, you type in the phrase "lung cancer treatment" using the Google search engine. Instead of possibly getting the Abramson Cancer Center at the University of Pennsylvania as your first result, you may get a 'sponsored link' from Aventis Pharmaceuticals, Inc. To their credit, Google does identify sponsored listings, but not every search engine is so forth coming.

MOTIVATORS

A medical site I visited recently reported that, according to 'the latest research', a certain diet that endorsed the liberal consumption of animal protein was extremely harmful to people and should not be undertaken. The feature story alluded to the irreversible harm that could be done by consuming so much fat. As there was no date on this story, an unsuspecting visitor to the Web site would assume it was current. It was not. Two larger studies that supported the diet claims had since been completed. Furthermore, upon investigating the supporting agencies of this particular Web site, I learned that there were close ties to a prominent animal rights organization. It would not be unreasonable to suspect, then, that the 'flavor' of the feature story might have been motivated by the agenda of the supporting organization.

THE SHAPE OF THE WEB

We have already talked about hypertext links, which when clicked on, will take you to an entirely different page of information. Now we will talk about how all of these pages are arranged and accessed.

FILE TYPES

Any Web page can include links to a number of different types of content. Clicking on the word 'enlarge' under a photo will pull up a larger photo, not a text or Web page. Hyperlinks can bring you to music, audio, video, Microsoft Word documents, and many other types of files. Many medical Web sites feature animations and three-dimensional (3-D) modeling to demonstrate drug interaction or biological processes. These file types include Microsoft's Media format, Real Video, Apple QuickTime, and Macromedia Flash, among others. Some text documents are converted to the Adobe Acrobat format (PDF) for more consistent viewing across various computer systems.

CONTENT

Content on a Web site is the stuff you actually see. It includes text and pictures and possibly links to the file types mentioned above.

Web pages can also retrieve content dynamically. A tiny code on a Web page can call on a database and present that data on the Web page as if it were part of the page. Databases usually contain information such as news stories or collections of similar data, e.g., a Web directory or membership list.

SEARCH ENGINES

Search engines are software tools that collect indexed information using "search bots" or "spiders" that continuously roam the Internet extracting data from Web servers and Web pages. The search engine attempts to arrange the collected data in some kind of logical order. This saved collection of Web pages (or "cached index") can be queried through a search form on the search engine site. Some search engines have developed simple methods for querying this data, but subsequent search results will include items and abstracts not related to your search. This is because Web-savvy marketers pay for search engine positioning based on specific keywords that potential customers are likely to use in their search.

While not all search engines allow pay-per-click positioning, the trend is growing. Search engines are becoming more a source of commercially motivated information than an efficient source of useful non-commercial knowledge. The good news is that much of the information we are seeking is catalogued in *directories*.

DIRECTORIES

The Web is constantly changing shape as new technologies are introduced and new content providers join the fray. Search engine bots 'spider' the Web quickly looking for changes in html pages and including them in search engine results almost immediately. The bots, however, are considerably less successful at cataloging databases or scrutinizing content for relevance or value. This is where directories are different.

Real people compile Web directories. Unlike search engines, which 'spider' or 'crawl' the Web looking for any and all content that is, technically, acceptable, directories are compiled by people who actually visit Web sites and manually review, catalog, and accept or reject Web pages for inclusion. Thus, the content of directories is much more valuable. It is also easier to navigate because you do not have to wade through gigabytes of unrelated information.

There are thousands of directories. For health content, specific subject directories are your best sources of reliable information. The main drawback, however, is that it may be a very long time before recent information is catalogued and made available. Two of the most popular general-purpose Web directories are Yahoo and the Open Directory Project.

THE INVISIBLE WEB

Most of the information on the Web is not available from search engines. Databases are, in fact, the primary repositories for most current information, especially new information that may change quickly or information that comes in the form of reports. Although there are some Web bots that try to access the content of databases, in general, search engines have a hard time searching and extracting such content. So it is best, especially for purposes of research, to access these primary information repositories directly rather than through a search engine.

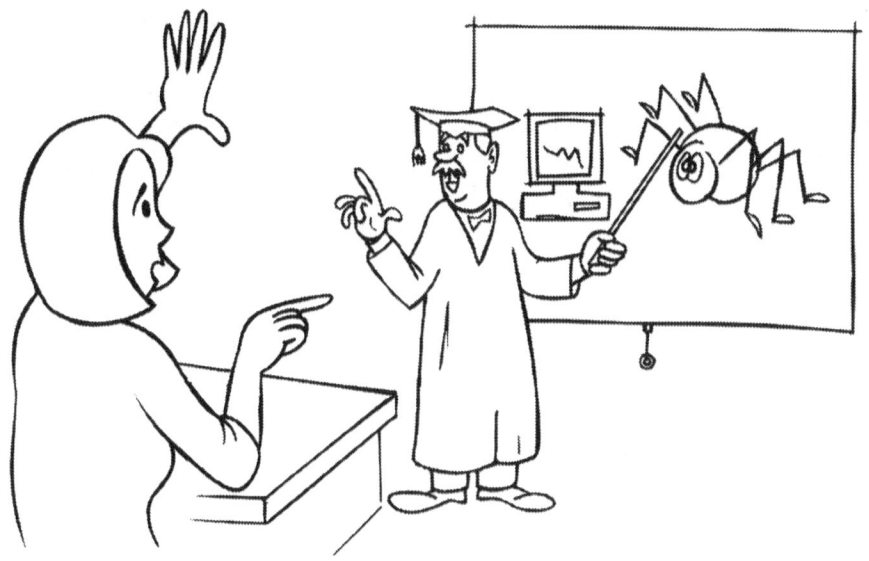

V. Search Basics

If you have not heard the term Boolean before, you are hearing it now. Boolean, Boolean, Boolean! Not to worry. The term is not as important or as intimidating as you might first suspect. A 19th century, self-taught scientist named, not surprisingly, Boole came up with a literary way of asking mathematical questions by simply using three words: AND, OR, and NOT.

Boolean logic is at the heart of most search software and it is pretty easy to grasp. Simply construct your search question in English and go from there. For example: "I want to learn about lung cancer AND treatment options NOT clinical trials OR press releases."

Each search engine, directory, or database has slightly different mechanisms for entering your question. READ THE HELP PAGE of each search engine you use. Try the advanced search form when you have the opportunity. Because much of the Boolean logic has already been applied behind the scenes, all you need to do is enter keywords, select a few parameters, and you are off and running. Some search engines will even let you search from within the results of your previous search, which is a big time saver.

Please note that this section is not meant to be a comprehensive tutorial on search engine algorithms. We have included links to excellent tutorials in the Appendix. Just keep in mind that search features change often. Understanding how each search engine works will not only enhance the accuracy of your research, but it will also save a great deal of time in the long run.

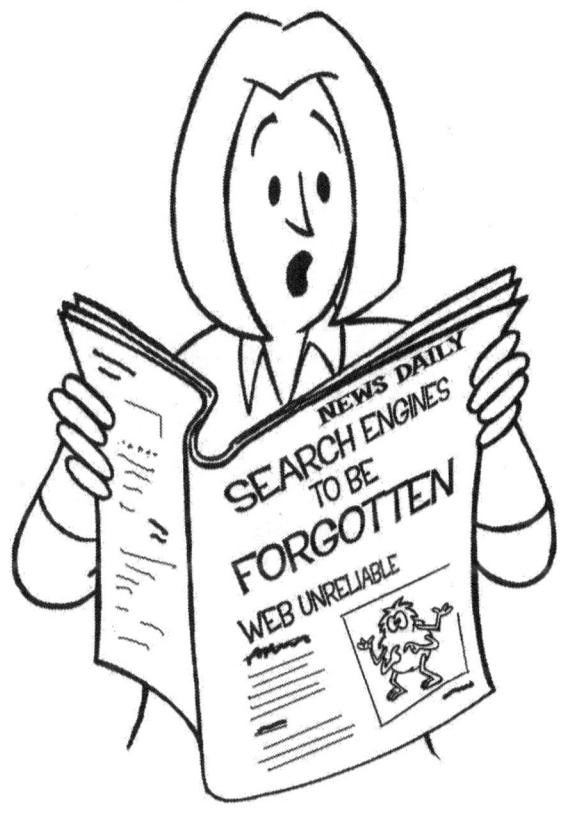

VI. Now, Forget About
Search Engines

Although search engines are amazing Internet tools that have a significant place in Web culture, they are not very useful for health-related research. In fact, to obtain the medical information you desire, you may want to forget about search engines.

To illustrate this point, do the following exercise. Type the word 'cancer' into Google's search form and you will receive millions of results. To get any relevant data from these results, a great deal of refining and filtering will be necessary. Now type in "non small cell lung cancer". Although the results are far fewer (about 250,000), it is still more than you will want to sift through.

Instead of narrowing the search, a search engine actually increases the number of potentially irrelevant results by increasing the number of sources of content, regardless of whether those sources are relevant to the search. Some of these results will be valid, but most will not, and finding all of the valid results will take more time than most of us are willing to spend.

While being familiar with the search engine you have selected is useful at the beginning of a search, it is a good idea not to depend too heavily on that familiarity. Use the search engine only to locate the real sources of medical information. If you read the rest of this book, you may not even need them for that.

Remember, the title of this book is *Searching the Web for Health*, not Searching the Web for Antique Bavarian Porcelain (in which case a search engine would be very useful).

According to a recent Pew report on health resources on the Internet, consumers go online to:

- Search for health information
- Research a diagnosis or prescription
- Prepare for surgery and learn more about the recovery process
- Get tips from other caregivers and patients about dealing with a particular symptom
- Give and receive emotional support
- Keep family and friends informed of a loved one's condition

*Source: Pew Research Center (http://people-press.org/)

The first three issues can only be addressed by large, well-funded organizations such as research institutes, hospitals, or university research centers. Many pharmaceutical companies also engage in drug research, while bioscience and genetics companies pour millions of dollars into developing new treatment options. Even so, there has yet to be an instance of an FDA approved drug being developed by a local pharmacy, nor has any neighborhood optometrist developed a new surgical procedure for an eye disease (although if you look hard enough, you might find one.) Yet search engine-based queries will include these types of information as well as thousands of personal health pages, and dubious sources of "new" pills, elixirs, dietary supplements, and pain relievers. The overwhelming majority of these Web pages and their content are of questionable origin and, therefore, not worth your time.

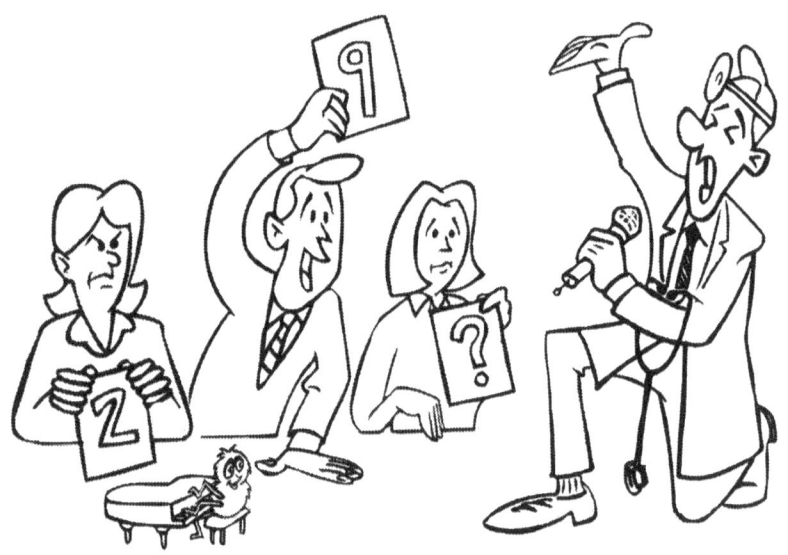

VII. Evaluating Health Information On The Web

Accidentally or intentionally misleading information provided during the sale or purchase of a house or car can be financially troublesome as well as a major inconvenience. Acting on erroneous medical advice, however, can be catastrophic. For this reason, extreme caution is crucial with any health information obtained on the Web. **Never act on any medical information from an online source without asking questions (additional research may be necessary to ensure that they are the right questions) and without consulting your own physician**.

WHO RUNS THE WEB SITE?

Knowing who runs a Web site can give you a clue as to its purpose. For example, a major pharmaceutical company may run a very informative health Web site. They want to appear credible, they need to be trusted, and in addition, they are being watched very closely by regulating authorities at a number of levels. Most of these companies will make sure to display corporate ownership information, names of editors, etc. On the other hand, a single individual reselling medical products may not feel the same pressure to accurately inform visitors of how the site is operated. So the rule for consumers is to make sure that there is an 'About Us' section on the Web site that adequately identifies the ownership of the site.

WHO PAYS OR HE WEB SITE?

While it may seem obvious that the owner pays for the Web site, this is not often the case. Webs sites cost money to maintain. Web sites can exist for a number of reasons, and each reason can introduce a different source of funding. Here are some examples

- Commercial Web sites – Funds are usually derived from advertising or subscription fees.

- Public service Web sites – Funding methods may include corporate sponsorships, and grants from both public and private non-profit organizations.

- Educational Web sites – Financial support may come directly from the school budget or from a variety of corporate and non-profit endowments

- Altruistic Web sites – In these cases, individuals or small groups usually pay for their own site.

Although valuable information may be found on each of these types of Web sites, for health research, the source(s) of Web site funding can be a concern, especially in terms of possible bias reflected in the information provided. The importance of knowing how and by whom a particular Web site is funded cannot be overstated.

Suppose, for example, that a single, well-intentioned cancer survivor, using his or her own money, sets up an altruistic Web site including a directory of cancer-related health information. That person may spend several weeks compiling links to interesting articles and other Web resources. As time passes, however, he or she may lose interest, become involved in other projects, or forget about the site entirely. The result is that the Web site is still out there with old out-of-date information still available to unsuspecting consumers. Another strong possibility is that the person who started the Web site did not have the professional training necessary to distinguish between relevant medical information and well-greased marketing materials. The bottom line is that the altruistic or low budget Web site often suffers from a lack of resources to ensure continuing high quality, up to date content.

WHAT IS THE ORIGINAL SOURCE OF THE INFORMATION ON THE WEB SITE?

If I told you that a cure for cancer was found last week, your first reaction would probably be "Where did you hear that?" Simply put, that is the same question you need to ask whenever you read about a new medical procedure or discovery on the Web. Reputable sites will always post the source of the material, often including a link back to the originator.

HOW IS INFORMATION REVIEWED BEFORE IT IS POSTED ON THE WEB SITE?

You may be surprised to learn that many of the news headlines you encounter on the Web are simply small pieces of code that call on databases to collect a predetermined number of headlines that match certain keyword criteria. In other words, there is not always someone who checks the source of the material for relevancy to the topic at hand. For medical information, human oversight is crucial and essential. Responsible Web sites use editors to select and evaluate relevant data. For medical Web sites, a person or often a group of people are specifically trained to separate marketing messages from reliable medical data.

YOU ARE NOT ALONE

There are several organizations that have been set up to address the problem of ensuring that the medical information provided on the Web is reliable. While their success rate is not 100 percent, they do provide a starting point for responsible Web publishing. It is hoped that this will evolve into a universal standard for health and medical Web sites. See Appendix for a list of the major players.

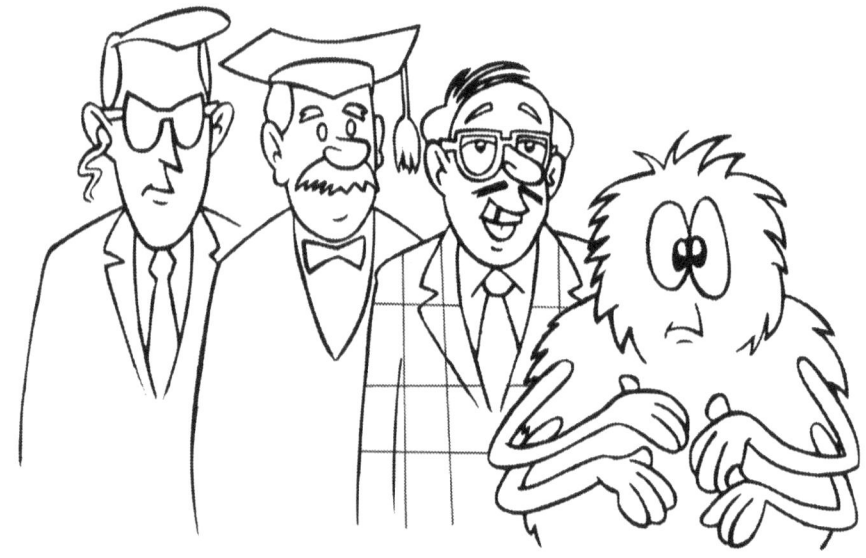

VIII. Reliable Sources

So far, we have explored the basic structure of the Internet, the rudimentary concepts of Web searching, and some of the technology involved. In the remainder of this book, we provide a list of the major sources of reliable medical information, along with information on how you can access these sources. This list **cannot be all-inclusive,** as we pay special attention to those institutions that are actively engaged in medical research today and that information is constantly changing.

The sources include government Web sites, academic Web sites, non-profit and public service sites developed by research institutes and hospitals, industry-sponsored sites from pharmaceutical companies, medical device manufacturers, and private research firms.

Other potential sources, which make a special effort to collect and archive information produced by the primary sources, are also listed. This group includes commercial health Web sites as well as the medical media.

THE US GOVERNMENT

All significant medical research has one thing in common: government participation in the form of regulation or funding, or often both. Consequently, the Federal government should be your first stop for health information. Most of the health information provided by the government will come through agencies of the Department of Health and Human Services (HHS). Through any of its major health information gateways, you can get information on clinical trials, research centers, medical devices, and background information on virtually all diseases and conditions. Below is a list of the more significant Federal sites.

FirstGov.gov

http://www.firstgov.gov/

With more than 186 million Web pages, FirstGov.gov is the gateway to every agency, database, publication, and policy that the federal government intends the public to see. FirstGov.com. is operated by the General Services Administration (GSA) The home page includes a welcome message from the President. Content is organized under four tabs.

While not specifically a medical or health site, FirstGov.gov can provide you with resources for Medicare and Medicaid as well as an ample supply of consumer education material. FirstGov.gov has been in operation since September of 2000.

One sub-site to note is FirstGov for Science. It is one of several portals into the health activities of the federal government. Be sure to check out this link. http://www.science.gov/browse/w_127.htm

National Library of Medicine (NLM) Gateway

http://gateway.nlm.nih.gov/

Developed by the Lister Hill National Center for Biomedical Communications (LHNCBC), the NLM Gateway is part of the National Institutes of Health (NIH). More than a health portal, the NLM Gateway is a meta search engine that will provide access to a number of "retrieval systems". (At the time of this writing, integration of the system was not yet complete.) From the NLM Gateway you will be able to search the following databases: MEDLINE/PubMed, OLDMEDLINE, AVs LOCATORplus, AVs LOCATORplus, ClinicalTrials.gov, DIRLINE, Meeting Abstracts and HSRProj.

Medlineplus

http://www.nlm.nih.gov/medlineplus/

Medlineplus is operated by the NLM and should be considered your first stop for any medical investigations. Working in cooperation with the NIH, Medlineplus provides one stop access to a wide range of health education and medical information services including medical literature databases, direct access to research studies through ClinicalTrials.gov, an illustrated medical encyclopedia, full text access to detailed drug information, a medical dictionary, and a large resource directory to help you locate hospitals, doctors, societies, nonprofit support groups, and other health resources.

PubMed

http://www.ncbi.nlm.nih.gov/entrez/query.fcgi?db=Pmc

PubMed is a cooperative effort of the National Center for Biotechnology Information (NCBI), the NLM, and the NIH. PubMed uses a search retrieval system called Entrez, which is also used by a number of other science databases. It is an extremely powerful text-based search engine that can access citations in medical journals. A feature called *Linkout* connects the user with the full articles of cooperating journal publishers. In addition, PubMed provides access to the Medline citation database of more than 4,500 journals from more than 70 countries.

ClinicalTrials.gov

http://www.clinicaltrials.gov/

Clinical trials are extremely important to medical research. They are required to determine whether or not a specific drug or treatment is safe and effective. Clinical trials are usually managed by the sponsoring agency, which can be a university, non-profit research center, the federal government or a private pharmaceutical company. ClincialTrials.gov exists to provide medical professionals and health consumers with access to clinical trial information. The site currently lists more than 8,000 clinical trials from more than 70 countries.

Participation in a clinical trial has advantages and responsibilities. It is an opportunity to contribute to the body of science that may lead to health benefits for many people. Each clinical trial listing a ClincialTrials.gov includes a summary of the study's purpose, the status of the study, whether it is accepting participants, the criteria for acceptance, and specific contact information.

On ClinicalTrials.gov, there are a number of ways to create a search query. You can browse through listings by disease, treatment, and location. Your best bet, however, is to use the 'focused search' option which provides a pre-formatted search form allowing you to quickly hone your search results.

TOXNET—Toxicology Data Network

http://toxnet.nlm.nih.gov/

Wouldn't it be great to have a single Web site where you could learn about the impact of various chemicals on our environment, our food, and our medicines? TOXNET is just that and more. An outgrowth of the NIH Toxicology and Environmental Health Information Program (TEHIP), TOXNET aggregates the data from a number of chemical databases under one Web site. The site includes links to consumer information, and tutorials bibliographies. It also integrates with the following databases.

- The Hazardous Substances Data Bank (HSDB) contains records on over 4,500 toxic or potentially toxic chemicals.

- TOXLINE®, with over 3 million entries, lays out the effects of drugs and other chemicals.

- ChemIDplus is the chemical database version of MeSH, providing nomenclature information to identify chemical substances cited in NLM databases.

- The Integrated Risk Information System (IRIS) includes Environmental Protection Agency (EPA) health risk assessment and regulatory information on over 500 chemicals.

- The Chemical Carcinogenesis Research Information System (CCRIS), sponsored by the National Cancer Institute (NCI) includes evaluated data and information derived from short-and long-term bioassays on over 8,000 chemicals.

Other accessible databases include the Toxic Chemical Release Inventory (TRI), GENE-TOX, a toxicity database of more than 3,000 chemicals created by the EPA y, and the Developmental and Reproductive Toxicology/Environmental Teratology Information Center Database (DART®/ETIC) covering toxicology literature collected since 1950.

Users may search all databases at once or individually. Additional resources are available including an extensive help system.

National Center for Biotechnology Information (NCBI)

http://www.ncbi.nlm.nih.gov/

The days of a single gray-bearded scientist working in a flask-filled basement laboratory are long gone. Today, computers, software, and large communications networks have become integral parts of the health landscape. From DNA sequencing to stem cell research, mountains of medical data require Herculean efforts to organize, track, and apply.

The NCBI is the government's hot bed of scientific discovery. The Web site opens on a rich collection of databases, tools, and resources that can help any serious student of medical research.

Home to PubMed Central, the NCBI Web site provides links to GenBank, a database of nucleotide sequences from more than 130,000 organisms, a number of molecular databases, genomes, literature databases, science tutorials, and a download area.

Genetics Home Reference

http://ghr.nlm.nih.gov/

This easy to use Web site provides information on genetic diseases and conditions caused by genetic disease. As of this writing, the site has cataloged 58 genes and 72 genetic conditions. The site also has a very comprehensible primer on genetic science, a genetic glossary, and links to additional genetic resources.

Genetics and Rare Diseases (GARD) Information Center

http://rarediseases.info.nih.gov/index.html

The NIH is offering healthcare professionals free assistance on two fronts in the form of its recently established GARD Information Center. Funded by the NIH's National Human Genome Research Institute (NHGRI) and the Office of Rare Diseases (ORD), the center provides healthcare professionals and their patients with immediate access to experienced information specialists who can furnish current and accurate information about more than 6,000 genetic and rare diseases.

According to the Web site administrators, the GARD Information Center was established in February 2002. Since then GARD has responded to nearly 4,000 inquiries on rare and genetic diseases. The requests include many queries from physicians, nurses and other healthcare professionals, as well as patients and their families who have been directed to the site by healthcare professionals.

Medical Subject Headings (MeSH)

http://www.nlm.nih.gov/mesh/meshhome.html

This is a helpful site if you are planning detailed research using PubMed.gov. The MeSH Web site does not have any articles, reports or other medical data per se, but it does provide a resource for using correct terminology to formulate your search. All of the citations used in Medline/PubMed are indexed according to MeSH standards.

Centers for Disease Control and Prevention (CDC)

http://www.cdc.gov/

The CDC is another mega-resource for health researchers. An HHS agency, the CDC is focused primarily on public health issues. On your first visit, you will notice an immediate emphasis on infectious and emerging disease. The pages offer a wealth of statistics on every health topic imaginable. CDCWonder, a search tool deployed on the site, allows visitors to query a large collection of reports, publications, and health data. While CDCWonder does have a registration option, like all federal health Web sites, it does not **require** any type of login or registration. Additionally, all services, Web pages, and online tools are available at no cost.

Food & Drug Administration (FDA)

http://www.fda.gov/

More than any other government agency, the FDA is directly involved in the regulation of those things that affect our health. Thus, the FDA Web site is a major source of health information. Here is a quotation from their Web site: "It's FDA's job to see that food is safe and wholesome; that cosmetics won't hurt us; that medicines and medical devices are safe and effective; and that radiation-emitting products are not harmful."

Like many other government agencies, the FDA has gone to great lengths to provide as much information as possible on its Web site. Although you may occasionally find yourself on a page that was last updated several years ago, the good news is that responses to questions are provided in fairly short order.

Make sure you visit the 'about' section of the FDA Web site. There is a free Web-based course that provides an excellent overview of the agency's activities and responsibilities, which are addressed through an organization of 'centers'. Below is a list of the most important centers related to consumer health issues.

Center for Drug Evaluation and Research (CDER)

http://www.fda.gov/cder/

The most important responsibility of the CDER is to monitor clinical trials. Their mission is to protect the rights of participants and maintain the integrity of the resulting data from those trials. CDER reviews the results of clinical trials and if the benefits outweigh the risks, they approve the drug.

The CDER Web site provides links to a number of useful resources including:

- The Electronic Orange Book – a valuable resource for obtaining patent information on pharmaceuticals

- The National Drug Code Directory – primarily a universal identifier mechanism for prescription drugs

- Consumer Resources – a well stocked shelf of electronic brochures and other consumer-oriented information about the safe use of drugs

- MedWatch – a service of the FDA designed to keep the public informed about safety alerts on medicines and medical products that have already entered the marketplace

Center for Devices and Radiological Health (CDRH)

http://www.fda.gov/cdrh/

Whether it is a drug or a new procedure, the process usually involves a delivery mechanism, which usually takes the form of a medical device. These devices fall under the jurisdiction of the CDRH. Medical devices play an important roll in diabetes, vision treatments, including LASIK, CT scanning, breast implants, and more. It is easy to see why the information provided on this site is so important.

Center for Biologics Evaluation and Research (CBER)

http://www.fda.gov/cber/

Through the CBER, the FDA addresses its responsibility for the safe supply of blood and blood products. The CBER is also involved in vaccines, allergens, genetic research, tissue transplantation, and host of other health-related biological activities.

Office of Special Health Issues (OSHI)

http://www.fda.gov/oashi/home.html

With primary focus on HIV/AIDS and cancer, OSHI provides a clearinghouse for medical information on these diseases. OSHI also offers a patient representative program through which patients and their families can provide a unique perspective to the FDA regarding specific diseases.

UNIVERSITIES, COLLEGES, AND SCHOOLS

Much of the cutting edge medicine you hear about on CNN and other news agencies originates from the public relations (PR) departments of major universities involved in medical research. All of us will be happy when a cure for diabetes or leukemia is found, but no one will be happier than the financial directors of the university that sponsored the research.

The gem of breakthrough research can indeed be found in the hallowed halls of many excellent university medical centers and research hospitals. The staff at most of these institutions is top notch, and most of their research is closely monitored by the federal government and the scientific community as a whole.

Occasionally, however, a university public relations department may release "breaking news" that was not yet ready to be "broken" to the public. For example, the *possibility* that a certain protein "may someday have an impact on the development of certain antibodies that could some day be used in potential treatments" is not the same as actually providing the new treatment. In fact, the treatment to which the story alludes may be years away from the clinical trials needed before it can be made available to the public. Bottom line? Read press releases very carefully.

Finally, when you visit these often eye-catching Web sites, keep in mind that they are, primarily, fund raising or student recruitment tools for the university. This is not to say that excellent health information may not be available on these sites, but rather that it is sometimes not easy to find.

HOSPITALS, RESEARCH INSTITUTES, AND NON-PROFIT ORGANIZATIONS

The hospitals, research institutes, and organizations named in the appendix are included because of their current level of research activity, It should also be noted that while each organization's perspective is often unique, none of entities operates in a vacuum. The government, schools, non-profit organizations, and the medical industry, itself, often work together in a variety of ways.

THE BIOSCIENCE INDUSTRY

As integral partners in the search for medical breakthroughs, private industry on the Web holds the key to a significant supply of both cutting-edge and archived medical knowledge.

Unfortunately, no where is the lack of publishing standards more apparent than on the Web sites of the pharmaceutical industry. While many sites do their best to provide helpful information to the visiting public, most are clearly selling specific products, promoting cultural or lifestyle perspectives that support their products, or attempting to raise capital for additional research. Although these activities are legitimate and necessary for any enterprise, the problem arises when the general public is intentionally under-informed or misdirected in the process.

If the pressure of marketing and PR can dramatically affect even the hallowed halls of our elite public universities, consider the impact of these elements on the overheated commercial world of drug development and genetic research.

Nevertheless, a discerning Web researcher can learn much about specific medicines and medical devices by perusing the manufacturer's Web pages.

SELECTED CONSUMER HEALTH AND MEDICAL WEB SITES

As we have attempted to show throughout this book, a little skepticism goes a long way when it comes to searching the Web. This is particularly true for commercial health Web sites, i.e., Web sites that in the business of delivering medical information for profit.

Unlike medical device manufacturers and pharmaceutical companies, who may provide consumer health information as an adjunct to the primary business of selling their product, or non-profit organizations, who may provide medical information as mandated by their mission statement, commercial health Web sites are motivated by profit, which usually comes from subscriptions, advertising revenue, or some combination of both. Web sites that offer subscription access to obtain higher quality information are, as a rule, more reliable than advertisement-sponsored sites. Reviewing each of the thousands of commercial Web sites on the Internet was impractical for the purposes of this book; we did, however, inspect several hundred of these sites and we have included them in the appendix.

THE MEDICAL PRESS

Intended primarily for journalists, online press services can provide up-to-the-minute coverage of breaking health news. The health science industry, while employing the skills and resources of major news services such as *Business Wire*, *Reuters* and others, has also spawned a medical media industry of its own. These services, though unregulated for the accuracy of the web site content, can provide a historical repository of developments surrounding specific diseases or treatments.

FREE HEALTH-RELATED 'ZINES', ELECTRONIC NEWSLETTERS AND E-ALERT SERVICES

Most, if not all, Web sites now include an invitation to subscribe to a free electronic newsletter or 'e-zine'. By the time you have scrolled through the glittered graphics and often questionable marketing messages, it is sometimes difficult to remember the source of the subscription.

Although health-related electronic newsletters may include the same sorts of dubious ads (e.g., diet pills, skin lotions, etc.), there are a few high-quality e-publications to keep you on top of this ever changing landscape.

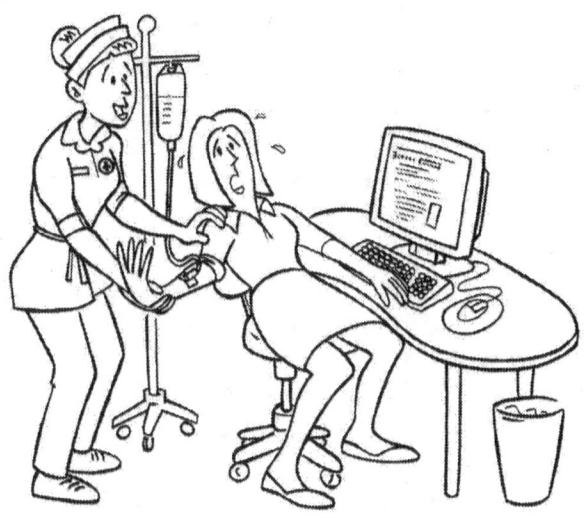

IX. Conclusion

When I started looking for health information on the Web, I knew that finding those nuggets of useful information that might improve our lives would not be simple. Marketing health products is one of this country's biggest industries and the well-fueled media frenzy that supports it is full of misinformation. Yet out there among all of the confusion, science does work and progress is made.

We could not dismiss medical claims by commercial companies as frivolous or misleading just because their Web sites did not end in *org.* or *edu.* It is important to acknowledge that thousands of companies in the healthcare industry spend billions of dollars on research and research-related activities looking for real solutions to real human problems.

On the flip side of this business politic, we also could not accept every health-related press release from every university PR department as the last word on health care.

Of course, if this was 1947 and I was 65 years old, none of this would matter to me. In those days, scientific discovery and application comfortably moved along at a seemingly sensible and timely pace. People "oohed" and "aahed" at the occasional discovery, but the biblical lifespan of 'four score and ten' remained the expected norm.

But it is not 1947, and breathtaking discoveries are happening all around us and at breakneck speed. Health claims that were considered sheer foolishness only a few years ago now receive serious attention from academia and industry alike. Medications developed only months ago keep people alive today while other medications significantly improve the quality of life for millions. As consumers, we speculate about the inherent possibilities of the increasing number of medical/scientific discoveries. With a growing sense of urgency, we ask ourselves: Can we live just a little longer?

Discovering the cure for a disease is a long and tedious process, but once it is done, the rest of us still must discover the discovery. Now may be the time to ask ourselves: Which of these is the bigger challenge? Our health and the health of future generations may depend on the answer.

Appendix

For Further Study

World Wide Web Consortium
http://www.w3.org/

Computer Industry Almanac
http://www.c-i-a.com

PEW Research Center
http://people-press.org

Welcome to the Web
http://www.teachingideas.co.uk/welcome

RECOMMENDED SEARCH ENGINES

AllTheWeb
http://www.alltheweb.com/

Google
http://www.google.com/

Teoma
http://www.teoma.com/

Alta Vista
http://www.altavista.com/

Surfwax
www.surfwax.com

Vivisimo.com
www.vivisimo.com

Ixquick
www.ixquick.com

RECOMMENDED DIRECTORIES

Librarians' Index
http://www.lii.org

Infomine
http://infomine.ucr.edu/

Academic Info
http://www.academicinfo.net/

About.com
http://www.about.com

Yahoo
http://www.yahoo.com

BUBL link
http://bubl.ac.uk/link/

The Open Directory Project
http://www.dmoz.org/

Complete Planet
http://www.completeplanet.com/

UCB Internet Resources by Subject
http://www.lib.berkeley.edu/Collections/acadtarg.html

Internet Scout Report
http://scout.wisc.edu/Reports/NSDL/LifeSci/Current/

WWW Virtual Library
http://www.vlib.org/

STANDARDS ORGANIZATIONS

The following agencies are involved in developing standards for the reliability of medical information on the Web.

Health On The Net Foundation (HonCode)
www.hon.ch

Internet Healthcare Coalition
www.ihealthcoalition.org/

DISCERN
http://www.discern.org.uk/

MedCircle
http://www.medcircle.org/

American Accreditation HealthCare Commission (URAC)
http://www.urac.org/

AMA Voluntary guidelines
http://www.ama-assn.org/ama/pub/category/1905.html#GUIDE

Journal of Medical Internet Research
http://www.jmir.org/

ACADEMIA

Schools listed below are actively involved in government-monitored clinical trials.

Arizona Medical Center
http://www.ahsc.arizona.edu/

Ball State University
http://www.bsu.edu/up/

Baylor College of Medicine
http://www.bcm.tmc.edu/

Beth Israel Deaconess Medical Center
http://www.bidmc.harvard.edu/home.asp

Boston University School of Medicine
http://www.bumc.bu.edu/

Brigham and Women's Hospital
http://www.brighamandwomens.org/

Brown University
http://www.brown.edu/

Case Western Reserve University
http://mediswww.meds.cwru.edu/default.asp

Charles R. Drew University of Medicine and Science
http://www.cdrewu.edu/

Columbia University
http://www.healthsciences.columbia.edu/

Comprehensive Cancer Center of Wake Forest University
http://www.wfubmc.edu/

Cornell University Medical College
http://www.med.cornell.edu/

Dana-Farber/Harvard Cancer Center
http://www.dfci.harvard.edu/

Duke Comprehensive Cancer Center
http://cancer.duke.edu/

Eastern Virginia Medical School
http://www.evms.edu/

Emory University
http://ww.medweb.emory.edu/MedWeb/default.htm

Fairview University Medical Center
http://www.fairview-university.fairview.org/

Fred Hutchinson Cancer Research Center
http://www.fhcrc.org/

George Washington University
http://www.gwu.edu/medical.html

Georgetown University
http://som.georgetown.edu/

Harvard School of Public Health
http://www.hsph.harvard.edu/

Indiana University
http://www.medicine.iu.edu/

Indiana University Cancer Center
http://iucc.iu.edu/

Indiana University School of Nursing
http://www.indiana.edu/~iubnurse/

Jefferson Medical College
http://www.jefferson.edu/jmc/home/index.cfm

Johns Hopkins University
http://www.hopkinsmedicine.org

Louisiana State University
http://www.lsumc.edu/

Loyola University
http://www.meddean.luc.edu/

Medical College of Wisconsin
http://www.mcw.edu/

Medical University of South Carolina
http://www.musc.edu/

New York Hospital—Cornell Medical Center
http://www.med.cornell.edu/

Northern Illinois University
http://www.gero.niu.edu/

Northwestern University
http://www.feinberg.northwestern.edu/

Oregon Health and Science University
http://www.ohsu.edu/

Rockefeller University
http://www.rockefeller.edu/research/areas.php

Stanford University
http://www.med.stanford.edu/

State University of New York
http://www.upstate.edu/

Staten Island University Hospital
http://www.siuh.edu/

University of Alabama, Birmingham
http://main.uab.edu

University of California, Los Angeles
http://www.medsch.ucla.edu/

University of California, San Diego
http://health.ucsd.edu/

University of California, San Francisco
http://www.ucsfhealth.org/

University of Chicago
http://www.uchicago.edu/uchi/resteach/groups.html

University of Chicago Cancer Research Center
http://www-uccrc.bsd.uchicago.edu/

University of Cincinnati
http://medcenter.uc.edu/

University of Colorado Cancer Center
http://www.uccc.info

University of Connecticut
http://www.uchc.edu/

University of Florida
http://www.health.ufl.edu/

University of Illinois
http://www.uic.edu/depts/mcam/index2.html

University of Iowa
http://www.uiowa.edu/homepage/hub/centers.html

University of Kansas
http://www.kumc.edu/

University of Kentucky
http://www.mc.uky.edu/

University of Maryland
http://www.hhp.umd.edu/

University of Maryland Greenebaum Cancer Center
http://www.umm.edu/cancer/

University of Massachusetts Medical Center
http://www.umassmed.edu/

University of Michigan
http://www.umich.edu/health_med.html

University of Michigan Comprehensive Cancer Center
http://www.cancer.med.umich.edu/

University of Minnesota
http://www1.umn.edu/twincities/07_health.php

University of Minnesota Cancer Center
http://www.cancer.umn.edu/

University of Nebraska
http://www.unmc.edu/

University of North Carolina
http://www.med.unc.edu/

University of Pennsylvania
http://www.upenn.edu/campus/health.php

University of Pittsburgh
http://www.upmc.com/

University of Pittsburgh Cancer Institute
http://www.upci.upmc.edu/

University of Rochester
http://www.urmc.rochester.edu/smd/

University of Southern California
http://www.usc.edu/

University of Texas
http://www.utmb.edu/

University of Utah
http://www.uuhsc.utah.edu/

University of Virginia
http://hsc.virginia.edu/

University of Washington
http://www.washington.edu/medicine/

University of Wisconsin Comprehensive Cancer Center
http://www.cancer.wisc.edu/

Vanderbilt University Medical Center
http://www.mc.vanderbilt.edu/

Wake Forest University
http://www.wfubmc.edu/school/

Washington University School of Medicine
http://medicine.wustl.edu/

Yale Cancer Center
http://info.med.yale.edu/ycc/

Yale University
http://www.yale.edu/medical/

ORGANIZATIONS

The organizations listed below are actively involved in medical research by either managing clinical trials, providing funding, or pursuing pure research.

AIDS Associated Malignancies Clinical Trials Consortium
http://www.amc.uab.edu/

Albert Einstein Cancer Research Center
http://www.aecom.yu.edu/cancer/new/default.htm

Alzheimer's Association
http://www.alz.org/

American College of Radiology Imaging Network
http://www.acrin.org/

American College of Surgeons
http://www.facs.org/

American Heart Association
http://www.americanheart.org

Anglo Celtic Cooperative Oncology Group
http://www.angloceltic.org.uk/

Arthritis Foundation
http://www.arthritis.org/

Barbara Ann Karmanos Cancer Institute
http://www.karmanos.org/

Beckman Research Institute
http://bricoh.coh.org/

Breast International Group
http://www.breastinternationalgroup.org/

British Columbia Cancer Agency
http://www.bccancer.bc.ca/default.htm

British National Lymphoma Investigation
http://www.bnli.ucl.ac.uk/

Burke Medical Research Institute
http://www.burke.org/

The Campbell Foundation
http://members.aol.com/campfound/

Canadian Institutes of Health Research
http://www.cihr-irsc.gc.ca/index.shtml

Cancer and Leukemia Group B
http://www.calgb.org/

Cancer Institute of New Jersey
http://www.cinj.org/

Cancer Research Institute of Contra Costa
http://www.cbcrp.org/research/PageInstitution.asp?institution_id=65

Carolinas Medical Center
http://www.carolinas.org/

Center for Medicinal Cannabis Research
http://www.cmcr.ucsd.edu/

Center for Molecular Medicine
http://www.molecularoncology.com/

Children's Hospital and Medical Center—Seattle
http://www.seattlechildrens.org/

Children's Hospital Boston
http://web1.tch.harvard.edu/

Children's Hospital Medical Center—Cincinnati
http://www.cincinnatichildrens.org/default.htm

Children's Hospital of Philadelphia
http://www.chop.edu/consumer/index.jsp

Children's Memorial Hospital, Chicago
http://www.childrensmemorial.org/

Children's National Medical Center
http://www.cnmcresearch.org/

Cleveland Clinic Cancer Center
http://www.clevelandclinic.org/

Cleveland Clinic Foundation Hospital
http://www.clevelandclinic.org/

Columbia Presbyterian Medical Center
http://www.nyp.org/

Comprehensive Cancer Center of Wake Forest University
http://www1.wfubmc.edu/cancer

Cook County Hospital
http://www.cchil.org/Cch/cook.htm

Cooperative International Neuromuscular Research Group
http://www.cnmcresearch.org/cinrg/index.asp

Crohn's and Colitis Foundation
http://www.ccfa.org/

Cystic Fibrosis Foundation
http://www.cff.org/

Earle A. Chiles Research Institute
http://www.providence.org/Oregon/Programs_and_Services/research/
e05chiles.htm

Eastern Cooperative Oncology Group
http://ecog.dfci.harvard.edu/

El Paso Cancer Treatment Center
http://www.accc-cancer.org/members/TX/mem670.html

Fox Chase Cancer Center
http://www.fccc.edu/

FRAXA Foundation
http://www.fraxa.org/

Fred Hutchinson Cancer Research Center
http://www.fhcrc.org/

Garden State Cancer Center
http://www.gscancer.org/default.asp

H. Lee Moffitt Cancer Center and Research Institute
http://www.moffitt.usf.edu/

HealthONE Alliance
http://www.health1.org/

Herbert Irving Comprehensive Cancer Center
http://www.ccc.columbia.edu/

Holden Comprehensive Cancer Center
http://www.uihealthcare.com/depts/cancercenter/

House Ear Institute
http://www.hei.org/welcome.htm

Huntsman Cancer Institute
http://www.hci.org/welcome.htm

Immune Tolerance Network
http://www.immunetolerance.org/

Institute for Drug Development
http://www.idd.org/

Institute for the Study of Aging
http://www.aging-institute.org/

International Breast Cancer Study Group
http://www.ibcsg.org/

James P. Wilmot Cancer Center
http://www.stronghealth.com/services/cancer/

Jonsson Comprehensive Cancer Center
http://www.cancer.mednet.ucla.edu/

Juvenile Diabetes Foundation International Islet Transplantation Center
http://www.jdrf-hms-islets.org/index.html

Juvenile Diabetes Research Foundation
http://www.jdf.org/

Kennedy Krieger Institute
http://www.kennedykrieger.org/

Kimmel Cancer Center (KCC)
http://www.kcc.tju.edu/

Leukemia Research Fund
http://dspace.dial.pipex.com/lrf-/

Lombardi Cancer Research Center
http://lombardi.georgetown.edu/

Long Island Jewish Medical Center
http://www.lij.edu/lij_homepage_ns.html

M.D. Anderson Cancer Center
http://www.mdanderson.org/

Massachusetts General Hospital
http://www.mgh.harvard.edu/

Massey Cancer Center
http://www.vcu.edu/mcc/

Mayo Clinic
http://www.mayo.edu/

Memorial Sloan-Kettering Cancer Center (MSKCC)
http://www.mskcc.org/mskcc/html/44.cfm

Mount Sinai Medical Center (MSMC)
http://www.mountsinaimedicalcenter.org/msh/msmc-home.jsp

Muscular Dystrophy Association (MDA)
http://www.mdausa.org/

National Cancer Institute of Canada
http://www.ncic.cancer.ca

National Cancer Research Institute (NCRI)
http://www.ncri.org.uk

National Gene Vector Laboratory
http://www.ngvl.org/

National Multiple Sclerosis Society
http://www.nmss.org/

National Surgical Adjuvant Breast and Bowel Project (NSABP)
http://www.nsabp.pitt.edu/

Neurologic AIDS Research Consortium (NARC)
http://www.neuro.wustl.edu/narc/

New England Medical Center
http://www.nemc.org/home/

New York Presbyterian Hospital
http://www.nyp.org/

Norris Cotton Cancer Center
http://www.cancer.dartmouth.edu/index.shtml

North American Brain Tumor Consortium
http://www.nabtc.org/

North Central Cancer Treatment Group
http://ncctg.mayo.edu/

Northwestern Memorial Hospital
http://www.nmh.org/

The Parkinson Study Group
http://www.parkinson-study-group.org/

Pediatric AIDS Foundation
http://www.pedaids.org/

Pediatric Brain Tumor Consortium
http://www.pbtc.org/

Rhode Island Hospital
http://www.lifespan.org/partners/rih/

Robert H. Lurie Cancer Center
http://www.cancer.northwestern.edu/index.html

Robert Wood Johnson Foundation
http://www.rwjf.org/index.jsp

Roger Williams Medical Center
http://www.rwmc.com/

Roswell Park Cancer Institute
http://www.roswellpark.org/

San Antonio Cancer Institute
http://www.ccc.saci.org/

Sidney Kimmel Cancer Center
http://www.skcc.org/

Simmons Cancer Center
http://www2.swmed.edu/cancerctr/

Southwest Oncology Group
http://swog.org/

St. Jude Children's Research Hospital
http://www.stjude.org/

St. Vincent Medical Center—Los Angeles
http://www.caohwy.com/m/md050502.htm

Sylvester Cancer Center
http://www.sylvester.org/

Texas Children's Cancer Center
http://www.txccc.org/

Texas Children's Hospital
http://www.texaschildrenshospital.org/

The Center for Science in the Public Interest
http://www.cspinet.org/

Tulane Cancer Center
http://www.som.tulane.edu/cancer/

University of Alabama Comprehensive Cancer Center
http://www.ccc.uab.edu/

University of North Carolina Lineberger Comprehensive Cancer Center
http://cancer.med.unc.edu/

Urological Research Foundation
http://www.usrf.org/index.shtml

Vanderbilt-Ingram Cancer Center
http://www.vicc.org/index.php

Washington Hospital Center
http://www.whcenter.org/

BIOSCIENCE INDUSTRY

The companies listed below are actively involved in current medical research and should not be overlooked in any search for reliable medical information.

Abbott Laboratories
http://abbott.com/

Abgenix
http://www.abgenix.com/

Acambis
http://www.acambis.com/

Acorda Therapeutics
http://www.acorda.com/

Active Biotech Research
http://www.activebiotech.com

Agouron Pharmaceuticals
http://www.agouron.com/

Alcon Research
http://www.alconlabs.com/

Alfacell
http://www.alfacell.com/

Allergan
http://www.allergan.com/site/

Allos Therapeutics
http://www.allos.com/

ALTANA Pharma
http://www.altanapharma.com/

American Medical Systems
http://www.visitams.com/patients/index.asp

Amgen
http://www.amgen.com/

Amylin Pharmaceuticals
http://www.amylin.com/default.cfm

Angiotech Pharmaceuticals
http://www.angiotech.com/

Antigenics
http://www.antigenics.com/

Ariad Pharmaceuticals
http://www.ariad.com/

AstraZeneca
http://www.astrazeneca-us.com/

Avanir Pharmaceuticals
http://www.avanir.com/

Aventis Pharmaceuticals
http://www.aventis.com/main/page.asp

Barr Laboratories
http://www.barrlabs.com/home.html

Bayer Corporation
http://www.pharma.bayer.com

BioCryst Pharmaceuticals
http://www.biocryst.com/

Biogen
http://www.biogen.com

Bioheart, Inc.
http://www.bioheartinc.com/

BioMedicines
http://www.biomedicinesinc.com/

Biomira Inc.
http://www.biomira.com/

BioNumerik Pharmaceuticals, Inc.
http://www.bionumerik.com/

Boehringer Ingelheim Pharmaceuticals
http://us.boehringer-ingelheim.com/

Bristol-Myers Squibb
http://www.bms.com

CancerVax Corporation
http://www.cancervax.com/

Cardio Vascular Genetic Engineering
http://www.cvge.com

Cardiome Pharma
http://www.cardiome.com

Catalyst Pharmaceutical Research
http://www.catalystpharm.com/

Celgene Corporation
http://www.celgene.com/

Cell Therapeutics
http://www.cticseattle.com/default.htm

Celsion
http://www.celsion.com/

Centocor
http://www.centocor.com

Cephalon
http://www.cephalon.com/

ChemGenex Therapeutics
http://www.chemgenex.com/

Chiron Corporation
http://www.chiron.com/

Chugai Pharma USA
http://www.chugaibio.com/

Coley Pharmaceutical Group
http://www.coleypharma.com/index_flat.html

CollaGenex Pharmaceuticals
http://www.collagenex.com/

Consultants in Neurology
http://www.cinltd.neurohub.net/

Corgentech
http://www.corgentech.com/

Corixa Corporation
http://www.corixa.com/

Cortex Pharmaceuticals
http://www.cortexpharm.com/

Cosmo Bioscience
http://www.cosmospa.it

Curacyte
http://www.curacyte.com

Cubist Pharmaceuticals
http://www.cubist.com/

Cytokine PharmaSciences
http://www.cytokinepharmasciences.com/

Daiichi Pharmaceuticals
http://www.daiichius.com/

Dendreon
http://www.dendreon.com

Discovery Laboratories
http://www.discoverylabs.com/

Dupont Pharmaceuticals
http://www1.dupont.com

DynPort Vaccine Company
http://www.dynport.com/

Eisai Medical Research Inc
http://www.eisai.com

Elan Pharmaceuticals
http://www.elan.com/

Eli Lilly and Company
http://www.lilly.com/

EMD Pharmaceuticals
http://www.emdpharmaceuticals.com/

Endovasc
http://www.endovasc.com/

Encysive
http://www.tbc.com/

EntreMed
http://www.entremed.com/

Enzon
http://www.enzon.com

Epeius Biotechnologies
http://www.epeiusbiotech.com/

Epimmune
http://www.epimmune.com

Eunoe
http://www.eunoe-inc.com/

Eximias Pharmaceutical
http://www.eximiaspharm.com/

Eyetech Pharmaceuticals
http://www.eyetk.com/

Fallon Clinic
http://www.fallon-clinic.com

Favrille
http://www.favrille.com

FeRx
http://www.ferx.com

Focus Surgery
http://www.focus-surgery.com

Fujisawa Healthcare, Inc.
http://www.fujisawa.com

Fujisawa Pharmaceutical
http://www.fujisawa.co.jp/english/

Genelabs Technologies
http://www.genelabs.com/

Genentech
http://www.gene.com

Genitope
http://www.genitope.com/

Genta
http://www.genta.com

GenVec
http://www.genvec.com/

Genzyme
http://www.genzyme.com/

Gilead Sciences
http://www.gilead.com

GlaxoSmithKline
http://www.gsk.com/

GTC Biotherapeutics
http://www.gtc-bio.com/

GTx
http://www.gtx.com/

Health Decisions
http://www.healthdec.com/

Hemispherx Biopharma
http://www.hemispherx.net/

Icagen
http://www.icagen.com

ICON Clinical Research
http://www.iconus.com/

ICOS
http://www.icos.com/

IDEC Pharmaceuticals
http://www.idecpharm.com/

Idenix Pharmaceuticals
http://www.idenix.com/

ILEX Oncology
http://www.ilexonc.com/

ImClone Systems
http://www.imclone.com/

Immunomedics, Inc.
http://www.immunomedics.com

INO Therapeutics
http://www.inotherapeutics.com/

Inspire Pharmaceuticals
http://www.inspirepharm.com/

InterMune Pharmaceuticals
http://www.intermune.com/wt/home

Intracel
http://www.intracel.com/

Introgen Therapeutics
http://www.introgen.com/

Isis Pharmaceuticals
http://www.isispharm.com/index.html

IVAX Research
http://www.ivax.com

Janssen Pharmaceutica
http://www.janssenpharmaceutica.be

Johnson & Johnson
http://www.jnj.com/

Kanglaite-USA
http://www.kanglaiteusa.com/

King Pharmaceuticals
http://www.kingpharm.com

Kos Pharmaceuticals
http://www.kospharm.com/

Kosan Biosciences
http://www.kosan.com/

KS Biomedix
http://www.ksbiomedix.com/

LEO Pharma
http://www.leo-pharma.com

Ligand Pharmaceuticals
http://www.ligand.com/

Lorus Therapeutics
http://www.lorusthera.com/

Maxim Pharmaceuticals
http://www.maxim.com/

Medarex
http://www.medarex.com

The Medicines Company
http://www.themedicinescompany.com/

Merck
http://www.merck.com/

Milkhaus Laboratory
http://www.milkhaus.com/

Millennium Pharmaceuticals
http://www.mlnm.com/

Millennix
http://www.millennix-inc.com/

Mitsubishi Pharma Corporation
http://www.m-pharma.co.jp/e/

Myogen
http://www.myogen.com/

Myriad Pharmaceuticals
http://www.myriad.com/

Nabi Biopharmaceuticals
http://www.nabi.com/

Neopharm
http://www.neophrm.com/

NeoRx Corporation
http://www.neorx.com/

Neurochem Inc.
http://www.neurochem.com/

NeurogesX
http://www.neurogesx.com/

NewBiotics
http://www.newbiotics.com/

Nitromed
http://www.nitromed.com/

Novacea
http://www.novacea.com/

Novartis Pharmaceuticals
http://www.novartis.com/

Novo Nordisk Pharmaceuticals
http://www.novo.dk/

Novogen
http://www.novogen.com/

Novuspharma
http://www.novuspharma.com/

Onyvax
http://www.onyvax.com/

Organon
http://www.organon.com

Orphan Medical
http://www.orphan.com/

Ortho Biotech
http://www.orthobiotech.com/

Ortho-McNeil Pharmaceutical
http://www.ortho-mcneil.com/

OSI Pharmaceuticals
http://www.osip.com/

Otsuka America Pharmaceutical
http://www.otsuka.com/

Pan American Laboratories
http://www.panamericanlabs.com/

Peptimmune
http://www.peptimmune.com/

Pfizer
http://www.pfizer.com/main.html

Pharmacyclics
http://www.pharmacyclics.com/

PharmaMar
http://www.pharmamar.es/en/about/

PharmaNet
http://www.pharmanet.com

Pharmasset
http://www.pharmasset.com

Pharmatech Oncology
http://www.pharmatech.com/

PhytoCeutica
http://www.phytoceutica.com/

Pro-Pharmaceuticals
http://www.pro-pharmaceuticals.com/

Procter & Gamble Pharmaceuticals
http://www.pg.com/main.jhtml

Progenics Pharmaceuticals
http://www.progenics.com/

Prologue Research
http://www.procro.com/

Protein Design Labs
http://www.pdl.com/wt/home.php3

QLT Inc
http://www.qltinc.com

Quintiles
http://www.quintiles.com/default.htm

Repligen Corporation
http://www.repligen.com/

Romark Laboratories L.C.
http://www.romarklabs.com

Schering-Plough
http://www.sch-plough.com

SciClone Pharmaceuticals
http://www.sciclone.com/

Scios
http://www.sciosinc.com/

Seattle Genetics
http://www.seattlegenetics.com/

Sepracor, Inc.
http://www.sepracor.com/

Sigma-Tau Research, Inc.
http://www.sigmatau.com/Research/Research.asp

SkyePharma
http://www.skyepharma.com/

Sonus Pharmaceuticals
http://www.sonuspharma.com/

Stressgen Biotechnologies
http://www.stressgen.com/

SuperGen
http://www.supergen.com/

Telik
http://www.telik.com/

Theradex
http://www.theradex.com/

Therakos
http://www.therakos.com/

Theravance
http://www.theravance.com

Titan Pharmaceuticals
http://www.titanpharm.com/

Transgene
http://www.transgene.fr/us/

TransMolecular
http://www.transmolecular.com/

Unimed Pharmaceuticals
http://www.unimed.com/

United Therapeutics
http://www.unither.com/

Unither Pharmaceuticals
http://www.unither.fr/english/presentation.php

Voyager Pharmaceutical Corporation
http://www.voyagerpharma.com/

Vical
http://www.vical.com/

Vion Pharmaceuticals
http://www.vionpharm.com/

Wellstat Therapeutics
http://www.wellstat.com/

Wyeth-Ayerst Research
http://www.wyeth.com/index.asp

Xcyte Therapies
http://www.xcytetherapies.com/

XOMA
http://www.xoma.com/

Yamanouchi Pharma America
http://www.yamanouchi.com/

ZymoGenetics
http://www.zymogenetics.com/

COMMERCIAL HEALTH WEB SITES

1UpHealth
http://www.1uphealth.com/

BioMedNet
http://www.bmn.com

BreakThrough Digest
http://breakthroughdigest.com

DiscoveryHealth.com
http://health.discovery.com

Doctor's Guide
http://www.docguide.com

eMedicine.com
http://www.emedicine.com/

HealthAtoZ
www.healthatoz.com

HealthWeb
http://www.healthweb.org

Harden Meta Directory of Internet Health Sources
http://www.lib.uiowa.edu/hardin/md/index.html

IntelliHealth
www.intellihealth.com

MedExplorer
www.medexplorer.com

Medscape
http://www.medscape.com

Merck Manual Online
http://www.merck.com/pubs/mmanual_home2

Patients Guide
www.patientsguide.com

Oncolink
www.oncolink.com

RxList
http://www.rxlist.com/

The World Health Organization
http://www.who.int/en/

WebMD
http://www.WebMd.com

THE MEDICAL PRESS

Health Behavior News Service
http://www.hbns.org/

IvanHoe
http://www.ivanhoe.com

Reuters Health
http://www.reutershealth.com/en/

EurekAlert
http://www.eurekalert.org/

Ascribe Livewire
http://www.ascribe.org/

Medical Newswire
http://medicalnewswire.com/index.shtml

FREE ELECTRONIC HEALTH NEWSLETTERS AND EMAIL SERVICES

BreakThrough Digest
http://breakthroughdigest.com/

Center for Drug Evaluation and Research
http://www.fda.gov/cder/cdernew/listserv.html

Center for Devices and Radiological Health
http://www.accessdata.fda.gov/scripts/cdrh/cfdocs/cfCDRHNew/listman.cfm

Dietary Supplements/Food Labeling Electronic Newsletter
http://www.foodsafety.gov/~dms/infonet.html

FDA Consumer
http://list.nih.gov/archives/fda-consumer-l.html

FDA HIV/AIDS
http://www.fda.gov/oashi/aids/email.html

FDA Patient Safety News
http://list.nih.gov/cgi-bin/wa?SUBED1=fda-psnews&A=1

FDA News Digest
http://list.nih.gov/archives/fda-newsdigest-l.html

Food Science (Nutrition)
http://www.cfsan.fda.gov/~dms/nutrsub.html

Food Science (Biology)
http://www.cfsan.fda.gov/~frf/biosub.html

Food Science (Chemistry)
http://vm.cfsan.fda.gov/~dms/chemsub.html

Harvard Health E-Newsletter
http://www.health.harvard.edu/hhp/publication/view.do?name=L

MedWatch
http://www.fda.gov/medwatch/new.htm

NLM Email Lists
http://www.nlm.nih.gov/listserv/emaillists.html

0-595-30343-9